MW01658521

Cookbook with

Succulent

Keto Recipes

Tasty Keto Recipes for You

By Alan Williams

© Copyright 2020 – Alan Williams - All rights reserved.

The content in this book may not be reproduced, duplicated or transmitted without direct written permission from the author or the publisher.

Under no circumstances will any blame or legal responsibility be held against the publisher or author for any direct or indirect damages, reparation, or m1tary loss due to the information contained in this book.

Legal Notice:

This book is copyright protected. This book is only for personal use. You cannot amend, distribute, sell, use, quote or paraphrase any part of the content of this book without the written consent of the author or publisher.

Disclaimer:

The information contained in this document is for educational and entertainment purposes only. We have made every effort to present accurate, up-to-date, reliable and complete information. No warranties of any kind are declared or implied. Readers acknowledge that the author is not engaged in the rendering of legal, financial, medical or professional advice. The content within this book has been derived from various sources. Please consult a licensed professional before attempting any techniques outlined in this book. By reading this document, the reader agrees that under no circumstances is the author responsible for any losses, direct or indirect, which are incurred as a result of the use of the information contained within this document, including, but not limited to, errors, omissions, or inaccuracies.

Table Of Content

CRANBERRY ALMOND MOUSSE

Ingredients

- 4 Tbsp cream cheese, original
- 28 g vanilla protein powder
- 1 cup liquid (produces 2 cups of whipped cream)
- ⅓ tsp almond extract
- 1 cup fresh blueberries
- ¼ cup sliced almonds

Instructions

1. Mix the cream cheese and protein powder with an electric mixer until mixture is smooth. Put aside.

2. In another bowl, beat the heavy cream with the almond extract until it doubles in size.

3. Gently add ⅓ of the whipped cream to the cream cheese mixture until the mixture is smooth. Add another third of the whipped cream by folding it into the mixture until it is well mixed. Add the 3rd end of the cream and fold until completely absorbed. Divide among 6 bowls, cover with plastic wrap and keep until ready to serve.

4. To roast the almonds, place them in a saucepan and roast for 3 to 5 min at 350° F. Sprinkle each bowl with cranberries and sliced almonds before serving.

Prep time:15 min; Servings: 6

Macros: 5.1 g net Carbs 4.9 g protein 20.4 g fat 1.9 g fiber

222.7 Cal

BLACKBERRY AND PEACH COMPOTE

Ingredients

- 4 fluid oz Sauvignon Blanc wine
- 2 Tbsp xylitol
- 1 tsp ginger
- 1 tsp cinnamon
- 3 medium-sized peaches (2-1 / 2 "in diameter) (about 4 per lb)
- 6 g of blackberries
- ½ tsp Thick-It-Up

Instructions

1. Combine wine, granulated sugar substitute, ginger, ground cinnamon, and peaches in a medium pan. Bring to a boil, reduce the heat and simmer for about 15 min.

2. Add blackberries and Thick-It-Up; continue on low heat for 5 min

3. Remove from heat and allow to cool to room temperature or serve hot. It can be chilled for up to 1 week.

Prep time:10 min; Servings: 12

Macros: 2.9 g net Carbs 0.4 g protein 0.1 g fat 3.3 g fiber 29.8 Cal

CARAMELIZED PEAR CAKE

Ingredients

- 2 Tbsp butter
- 2 Tbsp xylitol
- ¼ tsp ground cardamom
- 2 pears
- 3 large eggs (whole)
- 2 large egg yolks
- 2 cups heavy cream
- 2 Tbsp maple syrup (sugar-free)
- ½ oz liquid rum (without ice)
- 1 tsp vanilla extract

Instructions

1. Preheat the oven to 375° F.

2. Heat the butter, xylitol, and cardamom in a large skillet over medium heat. Cut the pears into ½ inch pieces. Once butter has melted, add the pears and caramelize for 4 min on each side. Remove from heat and place in a pie dish or 3-4 cup saucepan. Keep about 2 Tbsp syrup and pour the rest over the pears (keep the rest in the pan and set aside).

3. In a small bowl, beat the eggs, egg yolks, heavy cream, unsweetened syrup, rum, and vanilla in a combination. Pour mixture over pears and bake for 15-20 min until golden and the cream is hard. Remove from the oven and let cool slightly.

4. Brush the top with reserved caramel syrup with a pastry brush. When the sugar has hardened, heat it in the pan until it is liquid.

Prep time:10 min; Servings: 8

Macros: 7.2 g net Carbs 4.4 g protein 27.9 g fat 1.3 g fiber

310.2 Cal

HAZELNUT BISCOTTI

Ingredients

- 1 ½ cups chopped hazelnuts
- 1 cup whole flour
- 1 tsp cinnamon
- ¼ tsp salt
- ¼ cup sour cream (grown)
- 4 large eggs (whole)
- 12 Tbsp unsalted butter
- 3/4 cup sucralose sweetener
- ⅓ cup dried cherries, sugar-free

Instructions

1. Heat the oven to 350° F.

2. Finely chop 1 cup hazelnuts (reserve ½ cup chopped hazelnuts). Place in a small bowl and mix with soy flour, ground cinnamon and salt. Combine sour cream and eggs in a medium bowl.

3. In a large bowl, with an electric mixer on medium speed, beat the butter with the sugar substitute for 3 min until it is creamy.

4. Add half of the egg mixture, beat for 30 seconds, and scrape the sides of the bowl with a spatula. Repeat this with the rest of the egg mixture. Turn on the mixer at low temperature and add dry ingredients, mix until they are combined. Fold the cherries and hazelnuts into large chopped pieces. Let the dough cool for 1 hour.

5. Divide the dough in half. On ungreased baking sheets, mold each half of the mixture on a 12 x 2½ inch wooden block. Cook the logs for 30 min, until they are almost firm. Transfer to a wire rack to cool for 10 min.

6. Lower the oven temperature to 325° F. Carefully cut the logs crosswise with a saw blade into ½ width slices. Place the slices on baking sheets. Bake 17 to 20 min until firm and crisp. Cool the slices on baking sheets before storing them.

Prep time:45 min Servings: 10

Macros: 2.1 g net Carbs 2.4 g protein 7.5 g fat 0.8 g fiber 85.7 Cal

MINI CHOCOLATE LAYER PIES

Ingredients

- 2 ½ Tbsp Organic ground flax flour
- 2 tsp cocoa powder (sugar-free)
- A pinch of baking powder
- 1/16 tsp salt
- 1 oz Lily Sugar-Free Chocolate Chips
- 1 ½ Tbsp unsalted butter bar
- 1 Tbsp tap water
- 2 sour cream Tbsp (cultivated)
- 2 large eggs (whole)
- 1 tsp vanilla extract
- 3 Tbsp cream cheese
- 3/4 cup heavy cream

- 2/3 cup canned coconut cream
- 1 large yolk egg
- 2 Tbsp sucralose sweetener (sugar substitute)
- 6 Tbsp Torani sugar-free caramel flavor syrup

Instructions

For the pie

Preheat the oven to 350° F and set the grill to medium. Grease 6 wells of a muffin pan.

1. Combine flax flour, cocoa, baking powder, and salt in a small bowl; put aside.

2. Combine chocolate and butter in a medium-size microwave-proof bowl. Microwave in 30-second intervals, stirring at each interval until it melts; In total, about 3 min.

3. Beat the water, sour cream, ½ egg (beat an egg, divide the mixture in half, keep halFor the pie to add to the other berries), and ½ tsp vanilla. Add to the melted chocolate and stir until completely absorbed.

4. Add the flax mixture until it is combined. Spread the batter evenly over the 6 muffin trays.

Prep time:20 min; Servings: 2

Macros: 3.9 g net Carbs 5.3 g protein 27.9 g fat 2.4 g fiber

283.9 Cal

CHOCOLATE PUDDING

Ingredients

- 1 serving, plus milkshake with creamy milk chocolate
- 3/4 cup heavy cream, liquid
- ¼ cup erythritol
- 1 Tbsp cocoa powder
- 1 ½ tsp xanthan gum
- 1 tsp vanilla extract

Instructions

1. Use a blender to combine all the ingredients until they are well combined and thick (about 30 seconds).

2. For a large amount of ½ cup pudding into 4 separate cups, cover with plastic wrap and let cool in the refrigerator for an hour before serving.

Prep time:2 min; Servings: 2

Macros: 2.2 g of net Carbs 8.7 g of protein 17.9 g oFat 2.2 g oFiber 207.5 Cal.

CHOCOLATE BUTTERCREAM

Ingredients

- ⅓ cup heavy cream
- 2 oz baked chocolate squares
- 8 Tbsp unsalted butter
- ½ tsp vanilla extract
- 1 Tbsp cocoa powder (sugar-free)
- 6 packets of calorie-free sweeteners

Instructions

1. Heat the cream in the microwave until it boils (about 1 minute).

2. Pour over the chopped chocolate in a small bowl.

3. In a large bowl, beat the butter and sugar substitute with an electric mixer.

4. Add the cocoa powder, chocolate and vanilla then add melted chocolate.

5. Keep whisking until it is soft and fluffy.

Prep time:20 min; Servings: 4

Macros: 2.1 g net Carbs 1.4 g protein 19 g fat 1.4 g fiber 176.5 Cal

CHIA, CHOCOLATE AND COCONUT PUDDING

Ingredients

- 1 Generous Dark Chocolate Smoothie
- 4 Tbsp chia seeds
- ¼ cup coconut, grated, sugar-free

Instructions

1. In a medium-sized glass jar with a lid, mix all ingredients until well blended. Cover with a lid and leave in the refrigerator for at least 2 hours or overnight.

2. Cover with a pinch of cocoa beans), chopped almonds, or fresh whipped cream.

Prep time:5 min; Servings: 2

Macros: 2.4 g of net Carbs 7.6 g of protein 12.2 g oFat 7.5 g oFiber 175.3 of Cal

CHOCOLATE AND MINT CHEESECAKE BARS

Ingredients

- Bake 2 g of sugar-free chocolate squares
- 2 ¼ cups heavy cream
- ¼ cup unsalted butter bar
- ½ cup erythritol
- 2 tsp vanilla extract
- 2 large eggs (whole)
- 1 ⅓ cup tap water
- 1 3/4 cups sucralose sweetener (sugar substitute)
- ¼ cup cocoa powder (sugar-free)
- 1 cup blanched almond flour
- 1 ½ tsp of baking powder (straight phosphate, double effect)

- ½ tsp salt
- 1 pack of powdered gelatin (sugar-free)
- 16 g of cream cheese
- A pinch of of mint extract (mint)
- 8 Tbsp Hershey Unsweetened Chocolate Syrup

Instructions

1. Use erythritol powder (you need about ½ cup granules to make 1 cup powder). It can easily be sprayed in a blender. Measure it after it is in powder form.

Bottom layer:

2. Preheat an oven to 350° F and grease a 9 x 13 x 2-inch nonstick skillet; put aside. Melt the chocolate and ¼ cup heavy cream in a small bowl in the microwave 20 seconds apart. Once melted, stir to combine and set aside to cool.

3. Beat the butter and 1 cup erythritol powder in a blender for 5 min until it is soft and fluffy. Add the vanilla and the mixed eggs 1 by 1 for 30 seconds between each egg. Add the cooled chocolate mixture and beat until well blended. Add ⅓ cup water and ½ cup sucralose, beat for 1 minute.

4. In a small bowl, combine cocoa powder, almond flour, baking powder, and salt. Add to the dough and mix for 1

minute until everything is thoroughly mixed. Pour batter into prepared pan and bake for 20 min or until a center stick comes out clean. Let cool. Prepare the top layer during cooling.

Top layer:

5. Add the gelatin packet to 1 cup boiling water. Mix until all the gelatin dissolves, then place in the refrigerator for about 10 min (do not allow to stand completely, only cool to room temperature).

6. Beat the cream cheese in a medium bowl with 1 cup sucralose until it is thoroughly mixed and smooth. Add the mint extract and enough green coloring to reach the desired color depth (about ¼ tsp). Once the gelatin has thoroughly cooled, mix it with the cheese mixture.

7. Beat the remaining 2 cups of cream with the remaining ¼ cup sucralose until semi-rigid peaks form. Gently fold the cream into the cheese mixture until it is completely absorbed.

For this over the cooled brownie layer in the pan and leave in the refrigerator for 4 hours or overnight.

8. When they are ready to serve, cut them into 24 squares and cover with 1 tsp unsweetened chocolate syrup (Smucker's sugarless Sundae syrup works great because it is a little thicker than regular sugar). To make a spider web: start in the middle of the square to make a spiral. Take a toothpick and pull straight from the center to the outside edge. Repeat 5-6 times equally spaced.

Prep time:20 min; Servings: 12

Macros: 4.7 g net Carbs 4.9 g protein 20.8 g lipids 1.1 g fiber 219.8 Cal

CHOCOLATE MINT MOUSSE

Ingredients

- 1 ½ cups heavy cream
- 1 Tbsp chocolate whey protein
- ¼ tsp mint extract

Instructions

1. Beat the cream with an electric mixer until thickened.

2. Add the protein mixture and ¼ to ½ tsp mint extract.

3. Keep beating until it is smooth and firm. Divide into bowls and let cool 30 min.

Prep time:20 min; Servings: 5

Macros: 2.2 g net Carbs 13.7 g protein 22 g fat 0 g fiber 260.3 Cal

CHOCOLATE MOUSSE

Ingredients

- 7 g of unsweetened chocolate chips
- 1 ½ oz protein (dried)
- ½ cup tap water
- ¼ cup cocoa powder (sugar-free)
- 2 cups heavy cream
- 1 tsp dry coffee (instant powder)
- 1 tsp vanilla extract
- 2 Tbsp sucralose sweetener (sugar substitute)

Instructions

1. Melt the chocolate chips in a double kettle over medium heat (or in the microwave over medium heat for 1 to 2 min). Reserve and allow to cool to room temperature.

2. While the chocolate is cooling, beat 3 Tbsp dried white and water in a medium bowl with an electric mixer on medium speed, until the white is completely dissolved and firm peaks form about 5 min Put aside.

3. In a large bowl, combine cocoa powder with ½ cup cream, instant coffee, and vanilla until blended. Add the melted chocolate and set aside.

4. In another large bowl with an electric mixer, beat the remaining cream with a sugar substitute until semi-rigid peaks form for about 4 min Reserve 1 cup this sweet whipped cream (to cover) and incorporate the rest into the chocolate mixture in 2 additions.

5. Double the Protein in the chocolate cream mixture in 3 additions. Divide over 4 dessert glasses and cover with reserved whipped cream. Use a peeler to shave the remaining beautiful pieces of chocolate over the whipped cream if desired and serve.

Prep time:15 min; Servings: 4

Macros: s 9.7 g net Carbs 15.6 g protein 60.5 g fat 5.3 g fiber 714.5 Cal.

MINI CHEESECAKES WITH CHOCOLATE MOUSSE

Ingredients

- 3 oz squares of baking chocolate without sugar
- 16 g of cream cheese
- ½ cup sucralose sweetener (sugar substitute)
- 3 large eggs (whole)
- 3/4 cup heavy cream
- 3/4 tsp pure almond extract
- ½ tsp vanilla extract

Instructions

1. Heat the oven to 325° F.

2. Heat the chocolate in the microwave in 30-second steps until it completely melts; cool slightly.

3. In a large bowl beat the cream cheese on medium speed. Add the chocolate and beat until smooth. Add sugar substitute and beat until everything is mixed.

4. Add eggs 1 by 1 and beat well after each addition. Add the cream and almond and vanilla extracts and beat until smooth.

5. For the mixture into prepared cream cups. Carefully for boiling water into the pan to roast half of the mussels.

6. Bake in the oven until cheesecakes are puffed, and centers are ready for about 20 min Remove from the oven and let stand in a water bath for 10 min

7. Transfer the custard cups to a wire rack; cool to room temperature. Cool to very cold, 4 hours or overnight.

8. Garnish with mint sprigs, chocolate chips, and raspberries, if desired.

Prep time:10 min; Servings: 1

Macros: 5.2 g net Carbs 8.6 g protein 35.1 g fat 1.5 g fiber 362.5 Cal

CHOCOLATE MUDSLIDE

Ingredients

- 1 cup heavy cream
- 8 Tbsp Hershey Unsweetened Chocolate Syrup
- ½ cup tap water
- 3 Tbsp cocoa powder (sugar-free)
- 1 tsp vanilla extract

Instructions

1. Combine cream, ½ cup syrup, water, and cocoa powder in a medium saucepan.

2. Bring to medium heat.

3. Lower heat; Cook, occasionally stirring, for 5 min Remove from heat and add vanilla.

4. For the mixture into 2 ice cube trays. Freeze 2 hours.

5. Before serving, transfer the cubes to a food processor and mix until mixture is finely chopped and muddy.

6. Serve immediately.

Prep time:120 min

Macros: 7.6 g of net Carbs 2 g of protein 22.6 g oFat 1.3 g oFiber 232.6 Cal Cal

PEANUT BUTTER CHOCOLATE

Ingredients

- ½ cup Lily's Dark Chocolate Chips
- 2 Tbsp Lily's sugar-free chocolate chips
- 2 Tbsp peanut butter, creamy of course
- 3 drops of liquid stevia
- 1 pinch of salt

Instructions

1. Heat the dark chocolate chips for 30 seconds in a safe microwave bowl until they melt. Stir the chocolate and, if not completely melted, boil in the microwave at 10-second intervals and stop stirring between each until it is completely melted.

2. Bake the dark chocolate melted on a baking sheet covered with parchment in a uniform thin layer (1/8 inch thick).

3. Clean the microwave-safe container and heat the chocolate chips with milk in the microwave for 30 seconds or until it melts. Combine peanut butter, stevia drops and salt in melted milk chocolate chips in a combination.

4. Sprinkle the peanut butter mixture over the dark chocolate and use a skewer to shake the layers. Place in the refrigerator until it is firm, about 1 hour. Break into pieces and enjoy.

Prep time:10 min; Servings: 2

Macros: 3.3 g net Carbs 3.9 g protein 12.4 g fat 8.3 g fiber

126.3 Cal

CHOCOLATE CHIP COOKIES WITH PEANUT BUTTER

Ingredients

- 3/4 cup whole flour
- 1 Tbsp cocoa powder (sugar-free)
- 3/4 cup sweetener based on sucralose (sugar substitute)
- ¼ tsp salt
- ⅓ cup natural creamy peanut butter ⅓ less sodium and sugar
- ½ cup heavy cream
- 2 large eggs (whole)
- 1 tsp vanilla extract

Instructions

1. Heat the oven to 375° F. Lightly spray baking sheets with an oil spray.

2. Beat soy flour, cocoa powder, sugar substitute, and salt in a bowl. In another bowl, combine the peanut butter, cream, eggs, vanilla and chocolate extract (1 tsp; optional) until smooth. Add to dry ingredients; Stir until everything is mixed.

3. Place dough through Tbsp on greased baking sheets to form 18 cookies, 1 to 2 inches apart. Smooth the paste with your fingertips and flatten the cookies with a fork. Bake 8 to 10 min or until golden.

4. Let the cookies cool on the baking sheets for 1 minute before placing them on the racks so that they cool completely.

Prep time:15 min; Servings: 4

Macros: 2.6 g net Carbs 3.6 g protein 6.5 g fat 0.9 g fiber 86.5 Cal

FROZEN BANANA BITES

Ingredients:

- A cup of peanut butter

- One-third cup of toffee baking bits One oz. of

semisweet chocolate

- Four bananas (cut into rounds of one-inch thickness)

One tbsp. of shortening

Instructions

1. First, take a wax paper and cover the baking sheet.

2. Then, take each slice of banana and layer with one spoon of peanut butter. Take a toothpick and insert it through the banana piercing through the layer of peanut butter. Then, take the banana bites and arrange them nicely on the baking sheet. Freeze the preparation for at least thirty minutes or overnight.

3. Now, melt the chocolate and keep stirring it frequently. To avoid any form of scorching, use a spatula to scrape down the sides continuously.

4. Take another waxed paper to cover another baking sheet.

5. Take two to four bites of bananas from the freezer at a time and then use the chocolate mixture to coat them. Now, take the coated bites and place them on this baking sheet that you just covered with wax paper. On top of each coated banana, sprinkle some toffee bits. Do the same process with all the bites. Now, return the preparation into the freezer and keep it there for at least an hour. Before serving, keep the bites at room temperature for around ten to fifteen minutes.

Preparation Time: 20 minutes Servings: 48 bites

Cooking Time: 2 hours 15 minutes

Nutrition: Calories: 76 Protein: 1.8gFat: 5.1g Carbs: 6.9gFiber:

1g

ITALIAN KALE CHIPS

Ingredients:

- Four cups of kale (stems removed, loosely torn) One-

eighth tsp. each of

- Salt Pepper
- Garlic powder
- A quarter tsp. of Italian seasoning One tbsp. of olive oil
- Optional – One tbsp. of grated Parmesan cheese

Instructions

1. Set the temperature of the oven to 225 degrees Fahrenheit and preheat. The temperature of the oven is very important in this recipe; otherwise, your kale chips might just get burnt.

2. Now, it is time to prepare the kale. Tear the leaves and remove the stems. The leaves should be torn into bite-sized pieces.

3. Then, take a baking sheet and use cooking spray to coat it. After that, take the kale leaves and arrange them on the sheet in a single layer. Drizzle some more oil. Remember that too much oil can make the kale chips soggy, so be aware of how much oil you are using.

4. Now, take a small-sized bowl and in it, add garlic powder, Italian seasoning, pepper, and salt and mix them together. After mixing thoroughly, sprinkle this mixture evenly over the kale.

5. Once all of this is done, take the kale preparation and bake it for twelve minutes. After that, take them out, toss them a bit so that they get turned, and then return the preparation to the oven again. Bake for another five to ten minutes. By this time, the kale should be crispy. But keep a close eye on them since you don't want the burnt.

6. Once done, remove, and if you want, then sprinkle some grated Parmesan on top.

Preparation Time: 5 minutes Servings: 2 servings

Cooking Time: 15 minutes

Nutrition: Calories: 148 Protein: 6g Fat: 9g Carbs: 15g Fiber: 5g

APPLE AND QUINOA BARS

Ingredients:

- A quarter cup of peanut butter One cup each of
- Apple sauce (unsweetened) Coconut oil
- One tsp. of vanilla Half a tsp. each of Baking powder

Cinnamon

- Two eggs
- One and a half cups each of Rolled oats
- Quinoa (cooked and cooled)
- One apple (chopped after peeling)

Instructions

1. Set the temperature of the oven to 350 degrees

Fahrenheit and preheat.

2. Take a baking dish of 8 by 8 inches and coat it with oil.

After that, keep it aside.

3. Take a large-sized bowl and add the peanut butter, apple sauce, eggs, coconut oil, cinnamon, and vanilla in it and mix them all together.

4. Now, take the cooked quinoa and mix it too along with the baking powder and rolled oats. Keep mixing until everything is properly incorporated.

5. Then, fold the apple in.

6. After that, scoop out the mixture and spread it on the prepared baking dish. Make sure that it has covered every corner evenly.

7. Bake the preparation for about forty minutes. After it is done, a toothpick inserted should come out without anything on it.

8. Before you slice or store it, the bars should have cooled completely.

Preparation Time: 30 minutes Servings: 12 servings

Cooking Time: 1 hour

Nutrition: Calories: 230Protein: 7g Fat: 10gCarbs: 31g Fiber: 4g

AVOCADO TOAST

Ingredients:

- One garlic clove
- Four slices of bread (whole wheat variety) One tsp. of parsley (finely chopped)
- Juice of half a lemon One avocado
- To taste – Pepper and salt
- For toppings – One tsp. of hemp seeds and some olive oil

Instructions

1. Start by toasting the sliced of bread and use a toaster to do so. You can also do it on the stove. Once you have toasted them based on your preference, remove and place them on the plates.

2. Take the avocado and slice it in half. First, remove the pit and then use a spoon to scoop out the flesh of the

avocado. Take a small bowl and put the flesh in it. Then, season with pepper and salt and add the juice of half a lemon. Then, add the parsley.

3. Use a fork to make a creamy mash of the avocado mixture and make sure that all the ingredients have combined well.

4. Take the garlic clove and crush it with the help of a fork. Remove the peel and then take the inside of the garlic and rub it a bit on top of the toasts.

5. Then, scoop out the avocado mash you made and spread them evenly on the slices. If you want, you can sprinkle some hemp seeds on top and drizzle a bit of olive oil.

Preparation Time: 5 minutes Servings: 4 servings

Cooking Time: 5 minutes

Nutrition: Calories: 156.4 Protein: 5.1g Fat: 8g Carbs: 13.3g

Fiber: 4g

TUNA PROTEIN BOX

Ingredients:

- Four carrots (chopped and peeled) Four whole eggs
- One cup of grapes
- Two to three celery ribs (chopped nicely) One cup of blueberries
- Eight ounces of cubed cheese
- For the tuna salad:
- Two tbsps. each of Finely chopped celery Mayonnaise
- Five ounces of drained tuna Pepper and salt to taste

Instructions

1. Firstly, cook the eggs and make them hard-boiled.

Leave them to cool and then peel them.

2. Take all the ingredients of the tuna salad and stir them all together. Once done, divide the preparation among all the four meal prep containers.

3. Take all the other ingredients as well and divide them among the containers.

4. You can refrigerate the meal for up to four days if you refrigerate.

Preparation Time: 10 minutes Servings: 4 servings

Cooking Time: 20 minutes

Nutrition: Calories: 414 Protein: 27g Fat: 25g Carbs: 20g Fiber: 3g

PUFFED QUINOA BARS

Ingredients:

- Three cups of quinoa (puffed) Half a cup each of
- Nut butter Packed soft dates Non-dairy milk
- A quarter cup of cacao powder Half a tsp. each of
- Sea salt Cinnamon

Instructions

Take a square baking pan of 8 inches and then use parchment paper to line it properly. Take a large-sized mixing bowl and place the quinoa in it.

1. Put the nut butter and dates in a food processor and blend on high. Blend it so that the mixture becomes completely smooth. Then, add cacao, milk, salt, and cinnamon. Pulse again until everything has blended properly.

2. Then, add this mixture of dates into the quinoa puffs and keep mixing to ensure everything has combined well. Then, take this mixture and press it into the baking pan that you lined. Press it so that it is as even as possible.

3. Now, take the baking pan and place it in the freezer for at least half an hour. Then take it out and refrigerate for two to three hours. After that, cut it into squares (approximately 16).

Preparation Time: 15 minutes Servings: 16 servings

Cooking Time: 40 minutes

Nutrition: Calories: 98 Protein: 3g Fat: 4g Carbs: 13g Fiber: 2g

ROASTED BROCCOLI

Ingredients:

- Five tablespoons of olive oil or coconut oil

- Three broccoli crowns (sliced into bite-sized florets)

Two tablespoons each of

- Grated parmesan

- Lemon juice (freshly made) Four minced cloves of garlic

Pepper to taste

Instructions

1. Set the temperature of the oven to 425 degrees Fahrenheit and preheat.

2. Prepare the florets of broccoli by slicing them into appropriate size and then place them all in a bowl.

3. Use coconut oil or olive oil to toss the broccoli florets along with pepper, salt, and garlic.

4. Now, arrange the broccoli evenly on a baking sheet.

5. Roast the preparation for about twenty to fifteen minutes.

6. Once done, remove the preparation from the oven and then sprinkle some parmesan cheese and lime juice on top.

Preparation Time: 15 minutes Servings: 6 servings

Cooking Time: 30 minutes

Nutrition: Calories: 211 Protein: 9g Fat: 12g Carbs: 21g Fiber: 7g

TUNA PATTIES

Ingredients:

- Ten oz. of tuna
- One tbsp. of dried chives
- One-third cup of panko or breadcrumbs Half a tbsp. of

dried dill

- Two beaten eggs
- One tbsp. of Dijon mustard One tsp. of olive oil
- To taste – Pepper and salt Optional – lemon wedges

Instructions

1. Start by draining the tuna.

2. Then, take a large bowl and in it, add all the ingredients to mix them together.

3. Then, take the mixture to form four patties with your palm. Start by rolling then into balls and then shape them into patties.

4. Take a non-stick pan and heat the oil over medium flame. Add the patties and sauté them.

5. Cook each side of the patties for at least three to four minutes until they turn crisp and golden brown in color.

6. Take the lemon wedges and drizzle some juice on top of the patties.

Preparation Time: 5 minutes Servings: 2 servings

Cooking Time: 15 minutes

Nutrition: Calories: 249 Protein: 35g Fat: 8g Carbs: 8g Fiber: 1g

ROSEMARY KETO CRACKERS

Ingredients:

- ounces of almond flour
- Four tablespoons of hemp seeds
- One and two-thirds cup of parmesan cheese Half a teaspoon of onion powder
- Two tablespoons of rosemary (chopped) One ounce of butter
- Two large-sized eggs Half a teaspoon of salt

Instructions

1. Set the temperature of the oven to 375 degrees Fahrenheit and preheat.

2. In a mixing bowl, add all the dried ingredients. Whisk gently, but make sure that there are no lumps remaining.

3. Now, take a jug that is microwave-safe and place the butter in it. Melt the butter in the microwave. Add the eggs in this jug. Whisk the mixture until it becomes smooth.

4. Add this egg mixture onto the dry ingredients and mix thoroughly. A dough will form. At first, the dough can seem crumbly but keep pressing. Don't add any sort of liquids to the dough.

5. Keep the size of your over trays in mind and tear the baking paper accordingly. Now, take the dough and divide it in half. In case you are using smaller trays, divide it into quarters.

Form the dough in the shape of a ball and place it on the baking paper.

6. Take another sheet and cover the dough. Use your rolling pin to press the dough. The layer should be around 3 millimeters. Once you have rolled them evenly, use a knife to form the shapes.

Preparation Time: 25min Servings: 20(5 crackers each)

Cooking Time: 50 minutes

Nutrition: Calories: 111 Protein: 5.9g Fat: 9.2g Carbs: 1.2g Fiber: 1g

CROCKPOT PULLED PORK CHILI

Ingredients

- 2 lbs boneless pork
- 2 Tbsp brown sugar
- 1 tsp garlic powder
- 1 tsp salt
- 1 tsp pepper
- 1 tsp chili powder
- ½ tsp cumin
- ¼ tsp cayenne pepper
- 1 small red onion, diced
- 2 cups of beef broth
- 1 28-oz can of tomato sauce
- 1 can (28 g) of diced tomatoes

- ½ cup barbecue sauce
- 2 14-oz can bean with chili
- 1 tsp hot sauce, optional

Instructions

1. Place all ingredients in slow cooker.
2. Cover and cook 7-9 hours on low.
3. Remove and shred the pork roast with the forks.
4. Return to cooker slowly and combine to stir.

Prep time:10 min; Servings: 6

Macros: Cal 301 , Fat 7g, Net Carbs 2g, Protein 26g, Carbs 30g,

KETO MEAT BREAKFAST

Ingredients

- bacon slices, diced
- garlic cloves, peeled
- ½ onion
- cups of mushrooms
- 1 Tbsp fresh sage (about 5-6 leaves)
- 1 Tbsp fresh rosemary (about 1 large branch) 1 lb

ground beef

- 1 lb minced sausage (breakfast or Italian) 1 tsp salt
- 1 tsp pepper
- 2 eggs

Instructions

1 Cut the bacon into cubes and heat a pan over medium heat. Add the bacon to cook, stirring occasionally. Remove the bacon just when it starts to crisp around the edges, about 6-7 min Remove and place on a plate lined with paper towels.

2 Preheat the oven to 400° F. Lightly grease an 8x8 baking dish with butter or butter.

3 Put the garlic, onion, mushrooms, sage, and rosemary in a food processor. Treat until everything is cut into small pieces. Alternatively, you can cut everything by hand into small pieces.

4 Place the meat and sausage in a bowl. Add eggs, chopped vegetables, salt, pepper, and cooked bacon to the pan. Use your hands to mix the ingredients well.

5 Add the meatloaf mixture to the baking dish and spread evenly. Place in the oven to bake for 1 hour.

6 Remove and let cool at least 5 min before serving.

Prep time:20 min; Servings: 6

Macros: Cal 579 | Carbs 3g | Protein 31 g | Fat 48 g |

Saturated Fat 16 g

KETO PULLED PORK

Ingredients:

- 3 lbs boneless pork shoulder
- 1 Tbsp parsley
- 2 tsp cumin
- 2 garlic powder tsp
- 2 tsp onion powder
- 2 tsp salt
- 2 tsp bell pepper
- ½ cup beer

Instruction

1. Place all the seasonings in a small bowl.

2. Place the pork roast with the seasoned pasta in your slow cooker, skin side down, smother the roast completely.

3. Turn the roast to face the side of the skin. In the slow cooker, add the vinegar by pouring it to the side, no over the roast.

4. Place the lid and cook the roast on low or 8-9 hours on high for 10-12 hours.

5. Shred the roast when finished and put the meat back in the juice for 10- 15 minutes to rest. The pulled pork is going to absorb the juice flavors.

Prep time:5 min; Servings: 6-8

Macros: Cal 181 , Fat 8.3g, Net Carbs 0.1g, Protein 24.7g, Carbs 0.1g, fiber 0.05

SLOW COOKER PORK STEW WITH OYSTER MUSHROOMS

Ingredients:

- 2 Tbsp butter or coconut oil
- 1 medium onion, thinly sliced
- 1 clove garlic, minced
- 2 lbs pork away, cut into 1 "cubes and dried
- ½ tsp Himalayan salt
- ½ tsp freshly ground black pepper
- 2 Tbsp dried oregano
- 2 Tbsp dried mustard
- ½ tsp freshly ground the whole nutmeg
- 1 ½ cups bone broth
- 2 Tbsp white wine vinegar
- 2 lbs of oyster mushrooms

- ¼ cup whole coconut milk
- ¼ cup butter
- 3 Tbsp capers

Instructions

1. Add oil to a large pan over medium-high heat.

2. Add the onion and cook for 4-5 minutes, stirring frequently. Add mushrooms and cook 3-4 min more.

3. Sprinkle pork chops with paprika, garlic, salt, and pepper.

4. In the slow cooker, add mushrooms and mixture of onions, broth, and thyme sprigs to the pork chops.

Prep time:15 min; Servings: 4

Macros: Cal 611 , Fat 33g, Net Carbs 19g, Protein 63g, Carbs 20g, fiber 7g

KETO LASAGNA

Ingredients

- 1 lb ground beef
- ½ lb Italian sausage
- ¼ cup chopped white onion
- 1 ½ cups marinara sauce
- 3/4 tsp garlic powder, divided
- 1 tsp oregano, divided
- ½ cup ricotta cheese
- 1 cup grated mozzarella, divided
- 2/3 cup parmesan, divided
- Chopped parsley for garnish (optional)

Instructions

1. Preheat the oven to 400° F.

2. In a 12-inch cast-iron skillet (or similar oven-proof equivalent), brown the ground meat and the ground sausage over medium heat on the stove until it isn't pink (about 15 min). Drain off excess fat and heat again.

3. Put the onions in the pan and fry it with meat until it starts to soften for 3 to 5 min For the sauce, ½ tsp oregano and ½ tsp garlic powder into the pan with the meat sauce and simmer for 5 min

4. Combine ricotta, ½ cup mozzarella, and ⅓ cup parmesan in a medium bowl. Add a slight salt and pepper to taste and add the remaining oregano and garlic powder to the cheese mixture and fold until everything is well combined.

5. Turn off the heat and spread the meat over the pan until a uniform layer is left. Place the Tbsp the cheese mixture

around the pan, push them a little with your spoon at the bottom of the pan.

6. Sprinkle the top with the rest of the mozzarella and parmesan. Bake for 20 min until boiling, and the top begins to brown. Garnish with chopped parsley, if desired. Serve hot.

Prep time:15 min; Servings: 6

Macros: Cal 514.1 Fat 28.5g Carbs 4.9 Fiber .3g Protein 21.1g

COLLARD GREENS WITH BACON

Ingredients:

- thick-sliced bacon slices, cut crosswise into ½ inch pieces
- 1 small yellow onion, chopped
- 2 finely chopped garlic cloves
- 2 Tbsp sugar
- 1 tsp kosher salt
- ½ tsp freshly ground black pepper
- Spicy sauce from different scripts
- ¼ cup apple cider vinegar
- 2 lbs kale, without stems, cut into 3-inch-wide strips (or Swiss chard)
- 1 cup chicken broth (or water)

Instructions

1. Heat a high-sided pan with bacon fat or coconut oil while the bacon is cooking. Dice the onion over low-medium heat and add to the pan. Saute for about 5 min until soft. Add the garlic until fragrant for a minute, then add about half of the greens of the collar.

2. Before adding the remaining collard greens to the pan, let the collard greens wilt.

3. When done, remove the bacon on a towel-lined sheet of paper. Wait for a few minutes, then cut into small pieces. Combine the bacon with the wild greens mixture, then add in the apple cider vinegar.

4. Add the wilted collard greens mixture to a large slow cooker, along with 2 cups of stock. Cover them and cook on low for 5-6 hours.

Prep time:15 min; Servings: 4

Macros: Cal 72.9 , Fat 4.5g, Protein 3.1g, Carbs 6.8g, fiber 2.4g

CROCK POT LUAU PORK WITH CAULI RICE

Ingredients

- 3 lbs of roast pork
- slices of bacon, smoked nuts, and no nitrate.
- 1 ½ Tbsp Hawaiian black lava sea salt
- 6 garlic cloves, finely chopped
- 2 Tbsp free liquid nut smoke

Instructions

1. Set the crockpot to high setting and line the crockpot bottom with the slices of raw bacon. Sprinkle the garlic over the bacon.

2. Punch and stab holes all over and through the roast with a sharp knife.

3. Pour 1 ½ to 2 Tbsp black lava sea salt into a small pinch bowl and use your fingers to rub salt throughout the roast.

4. Place roast in the crockpot, fat side down. Add optional liquid smoke and cover crockpot over the top of the roast. Cook for 4 to 6 hours at high (longer bone-in roasting time), then for 2 hours at low. Could also cook for 8 hours to 10 hours at low (if your roast has a bone in it, it will take 8 to 10 hours).

5. Stir in the crockpot and cover shredded pork and bacon — Cook 30 min on low.

6. Steam cauliflower in the food processor for 20 min or microwave for 5 min, but slightly cooled cauliflower and add chicken broth, garlic, and sea salt.

7. Process until the texture of the rice is created.

8. Place a cauli rice scoop on a plate and add a shredded luau pork scoop.

Prep time:20 min; Servings: 10

Macros: Cal 182 , Fat 13g, Net Carbs 3g, Protein 14g, Carbs 2g,

Fiber 0.9g

CROCKPOT CHILI VERDE

Ingredients

- 3 Tbsp olive oil
- ½ cup chopped onion
- 2 finely chopped garlic cloves
- 3 lbs boneless pork shoulder, diced
- 2 cans (7 oz) green sauce
- 1 can (4 g) cut jalapeno peppers
- 1 can (14.5 g) diced tomatoes

Instructions

1. Heat the oil in a Dutch oven over medium heat. Saute the onion and garlic.

2. Add the pork and cook until the outside is browned. Add the green salsa, jalapeno peppers, and tomatoes in a slow cooker, and move the meat, onions, and garlic.

3. Cook for 3 hours on high. Reduce setting to low and cook 4 to 5 more hours.

Prep time:30 min; Servings: 12

Macros: Macros: 265 Cal; 12.4 g fat; 12.1 g Carbs; 22.5 g protein; 64 mg

CROCKPOT PORKLOIN

Ingredients

- 3 ½ to 4-lb tenderloin
- ½ tsp garlic powder
- ¼ tsp ground ginger
- A pinch of dried thyme
- Salt and freshly ground black pepper
- 1 Tbsp cooking oil
- 2 cups chicken broth
- 2 Tbsp fresh lemon juice
- 1 Tbsp soy sauce
- 3 Tbsp cornstarch

Instructions

1. Pour over the pork with the sauce. Close the cooker gradually.

2. Cook 4 to 5 hours on low.

3. Pork Shoulder-Cook for 10 hours on low.

4. Remove pork from a serving plate and cover with foil loosely (10-20 min rest).

5. Pour all the juices into a large saucepan in a slow cooker. Add the mixture of cornflour steam, blend.

6. Thickened sauce: Simmer for 5 min at medium-high or until it reduces to a consistency of syrup.

Prep time:10 min; Servings: 8

Macros: Cal 561 Carbs 28g Protein 56g Fat 23g Saturated Fat 11g

CROCKPOT KALUA PIG

Ingredients

- 1 (6 lbs) roast pork
- 1 ½ Tbsp Hawaiian sea salt
- 1 Tbsp liquid smoke aroma

Instructions

1. Pierce pork with a carving fork throughout. Rub salt over the meat and then smoke liquid. Place in a slow cooker.

2. Cover and cook for 16 to 20 hours on low, turning once during the cooking time.

3. Remove meat from slow cooker and shred, adding drippings to moisturize as needed.

Prep time:15 min; Servings: 12

Macros: 243 Cal; 14.7 g fat; 0 g Carbs; 25.9 g protein

SLOW COOKER ITALIAN PORK ROAST

Ingredients:

- 2 cans (15 oz) cannellini beans, drained, rinsed
- 1 cup thinly sliced yellow onions
- 1 red bell pepper, thinly sliced
- 1 Tbsp Italian herbs
- 2 vegetable oil Tbsp
- 2 tsp salt
- 2 ½ to 3 ½ lbs boneless roasted pork far, sliced
- 1 can (28 oz) Organic Roasted Cubed Tomatoes, drained
- 1 cup grated mozzarella cheese (4 oz)
- ¼ cup grated fresh basil leaves

Instructions

1. Pat the dry roast pork with towels of paper. Use a small sharp knife to make pork slits and insert the garlic slivers in the slits.

2. Use your hands to smash the leaves and mix them with the salt in a small bowl. Rub mixture into the nooks and crannies throughout the pork roast.

3. In the slow cooker, put the pork roast and cook on low for 14 to 16 hours. The slow cooker's pan will fill with liquid as the pork roasts.

4. It's fall-apart tender when the meat is finished roasting. You can shred it with forks, mix the crusty bits with the inside, tender bits, or break it into chunks of serving size.

Prep time:10 min; Servings: 4

Macros: Cal 130, Fat 4g, Carbs 3g Fiber 1g, Protein 20g

NEW MEXICO CARNE ADOVADA

Ingredients:

- 7 to 8 lbs of bone-in pork shoulder or back of pork, remove bone and visible fat, cut meat into 1 to 2-inch pieces
- 1 Tbsp. dripping with oil or bacon
- ½ medium onion
- 4-6 large garlic cloves
- 25-30 pods of red pepper, without stems or seeds. Pods cut in lengths of 1 to 2 inches
- 1 tsp salt
- 2 tsp Mexican oregano
- 3 cups of water
- 2 medium red chili powder tsp (optional)
- 1 tsp honey (optional)

- 2 tsp apple cider vinegar

Instructions

1. Remove from the red chiles the stems and seeds. Cut into 1" strips.

2. Add olive oil over medium heat to a large saucepan. Mix in chilies, onions, and garlic. Saute for 5 to 10 min until fragrant. Pour in milk, salt, and oregano, stirring well.

3. Bring to a boil, cover, and reduce heat to a simmer for 10 min.

4. Move chili mixture to a blender, in batches if needed, and mix until smooth.

Prep time:60 min; Servings: 4

Macros: 704 Cal 38g Fat 26g Carbs 63g Protein

PULLED PORK TACO SALAD

Ingredients:

- 1 batch of slow cooking pork extract
- 2 cups grated romaine lettuce
- 1 2-minute batch of pico de gallo
- 1 lot of guacamole
- 1 red bell pepper, seedless and sliced
- ½ white or red onions, sliced
- 1 Tbsp main flavor marinade herbs
- 1 Tbsp avocado oil
- Dressing of your choice

Instructions

Heat avocado oil over medium-high heat in a casserole dish.

1. Add the peppers and onions sliced, and the seasoning with adobo.

2. Cut the onions and peppers until they are relatively soft but not mushy.

3. Place shredded lettuce with pulled pork, guacamole, pico de gallo, and onion and pepper mixture in a bowl and top.

4. Top with dressing of choice.

Prep time:10 min; Servings: 4

Macros: 934 Cal, 83g Carbs 70g Fat, 41g Protein

SLOW COOKER COCONUT CURRY PORK

Ingredients:

- 2 Tbsp vegetable oil
- 4-lb boneless pork shoulder, cut into 2-inch pieces
- Salt and freshly ground pepper
- 1 large onion, minced
- 3 garlic cloves, finely chopped
- 3 Tbsp chopped fresh ginger
- 1 Tbsp mild curry powder
- 1 Tbsp ground cumin
- ½ tsp ground turmeric
- A 14-oz can of tomato cubes
- 1 cup unsweetened coconut milk
- 3 cups chicken broth or low sodium broth

- Steamed rice, chopped cilantro, and sliced new onions, for serving

Instruction

1. Heat the oil in a large skillet. Spice the salt and peppered pork and add half of the pork to the skillet and brown over moderately high heat for about 12 min
2. Put the pork in the slow cooker. Repeat the rest of the pig.
3. Pour off the fat in the skillet except for 2 tsp.
4. Add the onion, curry, cumin, garlic, ginger, and turmeric and cook until the onion is softened for about 5 min Scrape into the slow cooker the mixture.
5. Add the coconut milk, tomatoes and their juices, stock cover, and cook for 4 hours on high.
6. Spoon off much fat as possible from the stew's surface.

Prep time:15 min; Servings: 4

Macros: Cal 457, Fat 32.0 g, Saturated 15.9 g Carbs21.9 g Fiber 2.6 g Sugar1.7 g Protein 22.1 g

KETO SLOW COOKER BRISKET CHILI

Ingredients

- 1.5 lb beef (675 g), (boneless)
- 2 Tbsp olive oil
- 1 onion, peeled and finely chopped
- 2 garlic cloves, peeled and chopped
- 9 oz mushrooms, sliced (255 g)
- 1 green pepper, seedless and finely chopped
- 1 jalapeño pepper, seedless and chopped (optional)
- 2 Tbsp (12 g) ground cumin
- 1 Tbsp (6 g) chili powder
- 2 cups (480 mL) beef broth
- 1 can of tomato cubes (400 g)
- Salt and freshly ground black pepper

- Flat-leaf parsley or sliced jalapeño pepper for garnish (optional)

Instructions

1. Heat olive oil in a big pan. Brown beef and conserve liquid broth.
2. Add onion, garlic, mushrooms, green pepper, and jalapeno pepper.
3. Add cumin powder and chili powder.
4. Place the beef with fried vegetables in a slow cooker. Add the meat broth and tomatoes. Cover and cook for 6 hours at medium temperature, turning regularly.
5. Puree the meat in the slow cooker and cook another hour.
6. Serve on mashed cauliflower with salt and freshly ground black pepper.

Prep time:15 min; Servings: 6

Macros: Cal 43, Sugar 4g, Fat 3g, Carbs 8g, Fiber 2g, Protein 22

g

KETO CROCKPOT BEEF STROGANOFF

Ingredients

- 1 onion, sliced and quartered
- 2 crushed garlic cloves
- 2 diced bacon slices
- 500 g veal, diced beeFillet
- 1 tsp smoked pepper
- 3 Tbsp tomato puree
- 250 ml beef broth
- 250 g quartered mushrooms

Instructions

1. In a slow cooker/crockpot, place the beef, onion, garlic, mushrooms, beef broth, black pepper, and salt and cook at a low temperature for 6 to 8 hours.

2. Stir in coconut cream, Dijon mustard, salt to taste after the beef has been cooked.

3. Place the noodles of the cucumber in a bowl. Top with the stroganoff beef. Garnish with parsley.

Prep time:10 min; Servings: 6

Macros: Cal 462 Sugar 2g Saturated Fat 36g Carbs 4g Fiber 1 g Protein 26 g

CPSIA information can be obtained
at www.ICGtesting.com
Printed in the USA
LVHW080837260421
685568LV00005B/403

9 781802 327793